Weight Training For Results

How to Optimize Your Weight Lifting and Athletic Performance as Fast as Possible

This book is solely for information and educational purposes and is not medical advice. Please consult a medical or health professional before you begin any exercise, nutrition, or supplementation program or if you have questions about your health.

ISBN: 9781720134831

TABLE OF CONTENTS

Introduction: Working Smarter

Would you rather work hard or work smart? I feel both are necessary to achieve greatness, but you can't go far without one or the other. From my perspective, I envision that the end goal is whatever someone is trying to achieve (their goal), which is a pointer to a destination on a map. Working smart is like setting up the compass to go in the right direction, while working hard is actually doing the driving. You won't go anywhere if you don't work hard, and you'll go the wrong way if you only work hard, because you were not working smart to be able to go in the right direction. However, you might reach your final destination the fastest, if you point the compass in the right direction and move quickly by **simultaneously working smart and hard.** Since you are reading this book, you are probably a hard worker, and this book will supplement your efforts by having you reach your goals in the fastest way possible.

There are many reasons to weight lift. Weight training reduces stress, decreases the risk of injury (for sports and in general), it improves posture, longevity, as well as improve athletic performance. However, not everyone has the time to spend 2 hours in the gym 6 days a week for various reasons such as school, work, social events, sports, and family. In this book, you will learn how to lift based off desired goals, how to periodize your training, and how to optimize your performance; all in as little time as possible. Through reading, you will become better at working smarter; pointing the compass in the right direction.

Phases of Weight Training For Athletes

Some weight lifting coaches and common sports weight lifting programs do not periodize their weight training program. For optimal sport and strength performance, periodizing your training is a great way to get a competitive edge. There are 5 main phases for a weight training program. Generally, the program should last a few months to a year, but is a great fit for a season's worth of time (3-6 months for most sports). **The 5 phases are:**

1. Hypertrophy

2. Basic Strength

3. Strength and Power

4. Taper

5. Active Rest

Phase One: Hypertrophy

During this phase, the athlete is getting adjusted to the weights due to a prolonged break, even if it's their first time of weight lifting. Even experienced lifters should start this phase if they are starting a new athletic season or just want to hit the "reset button" on achieving new muscle gains. The goal of this phase is to add a bit more muscle to their frame and achieve **nuclei overload**. The nuclei overload is basically adapting the muscles for more *potential* future growth and strength, by keeping a constant stress on your muscles.

This is another reason why athletes that started while young are better prepared to be exceptional athletes when older; they had extra overload of their muscle nuclei from exercising in their youth. However, don't be worried if you did not play sports when you were a kid; you can incorporate this training at any time and achieve superior results when done properly.

Remember, the more muscle that is built in this phase, the more potential for future strength.

A great protocol for the hypertrophy phase is to focus on high volume but low intensity training. This means around **3-5 sets of an exercise with 8-15+ reps**, to build up your nuclei. The more days of the week the athlete lifts (frequency), the more volume they can achieve. This period's length will depend on how much the athlete has trained, and should last a bit longer for newer lifters. This period is usually 2-6 weeks.

The 300 Rep Challenge

After my first swim season in college, my friend, Gabe and I decided to lift for the first time after weeks of tapering in swimming. As we were finishing up our training, we ran into our lifting coach from the season, Parker. "You guys wanna do some biceps with me before you leave?" he asked.

Gabe and I looked at each other and exclaimed, "Yeah sounds great!"

Parker replied, "Okay we're going to do some bicep blasters!" "What are bicep blasters?" we asked. "We're going to do a total of 300 reps of bicep curls, starting with the heaviest barbell. Once you fail at the highest weight, immediately drop to the next highest weight and go until failure. Count your reps and you can't stop until you reach 300. No rest," he said with a maniacal grin and tone.

Gabe started with the 100 pound barbell (he's pretty strong), and I started with the 90 pound barbell. We did as we were told and after a few reps, we dropped the weight. After around 50 reps, we had to rest (with a little bit of ridicule from Parker). After 100 reps, we had to move to dumbbell curls (DB). At around 250 reps, we had to rest after performing just 5 reps of 5 pounds! It is noteworthy to state that the three of us finished the 300 reps, with our biceps "blasted". However, the next day in class, we could not even lift our pencils to take notes, because our biceps were so sore!

This anecdote is an extreme example of hypertrophy type training, but even more exemplifies the nuclei overload of the muscle. Since then, I have barely trained biceps no more than once every two weeks. My biceps have hardly shrunk since then, and they respond exceptionally well to any training stimulus. It just follows back to the principal that the more reps, sets, and days you exercise, the more *future* potential for strength and muscle retention. If you are just starting out or have taken a break for a while, the more reps, sets, and times per week you lift, the better off you will be by the end of your program. From my own opinion and for quick reminder, think,

"Volume, Volume, Volume!" (Volume=SETS X REPS X FREQUENCY).

Phase Two: Basic Strength

The main focus of Basic Strength is how it sounds, building strength. Since the athlete is to focus on strength, the rep ranges have to decrease with the actual weights increasing. Typical Basic Strength programs fall under 3-5 sets of 5 reps, with 5X5 being very popular. This period is a transition from high volume to medium volume, but bringing up the intensity to the next level. This period usually lasts 3-4 weeks. This is the transitional period from hypertrophy to total strength and power.

Phase Three: Strength and Power

In this phase, gaining strength and not size is the goal. If you are training for a sport, you don't want too much muscle on your frame as it may hinder some speed, so growth should start slowing down at this point to create time to focus on strength. Going through these phases properly will help you in the long term by *resensitizing* your body for future hypertrophy phases to come. Strength training phases and programs increase the maximum tension your muscle fibers can handle, which will translate to faster speeds in one's sport.

To increase the strength of an athlete, reps have to be lowered further. This phase is also a time to begin building power in the athlete; lifting not only with more weight but more *speed*. To gain power, an athlete must decrease the volume of training to be able to recover and become more explosive through safe, controlled movements.

Sets in this phase are generally between 3 and 5, while reps go down further to 1-3 reps per set. This phase lasts anywhere from 2-4 weeks, depending on the season length of the sport. For example, if your season lasts 6 months, this phase should last 4 weeks. If your season is 3 months, this phase should last around 2 weeks.

Phase Four: Tapering

Tapering or "peaking" is the phase that athletes tend to love the most. This is when the athlete should receive massive amounts of rest, with most of the volume cut down. The goal of this phase is to get the athlete used to **exerting maximum force** into the weights, benefiting greatly from lots of rest. Rep ranges in this period are still between 1-3, but the *volume* drops to as little as 1-3 sets per session.

Fun Fact: The Russian Olympic Weightlifting team loves doing **5 sets of 2 reps**

3x per week is optimal during this period lasting 1-3 weeks. After tapering, an athlete should feel very energetic, powerful, and ready for their max lift or competition.

How Long to Taper?

A difficult question to answer for weightlifters and athletes all around is, "How long should I taper for?"

This question is asked because if you taper for too long, you "miss your taper" and your muscles and body become deconditioned through not enough stimulus. This will lead to poor performance at your final max lifts (or sports competition).

On the flip side, if your taper is not long enough, your body will be too broken down and your body has not recovered in time for your competition, also leading to poor results. While it's hard to tell *exactly* how long you need, there are a few guidelines you can follow.

- **Body Fat %**: If you tend to have a low body fat percentage (under 12% for men and 22% for women), you will need a **longer taper.**

- **Muscle Mass**: If you have a lot of physical muscle mass built up, you will need a **longer taper,** since there is more muscle that needs recovery compared to an average person.
- **How you feel**: It's okay to listen to your body. If you are rundown and extremely more tired than usual by the time you reach the taper portion, you will need a **longer taper.**

It is important to be aware of these factors as taper is a **highly individualized** time period where the athlete has to be truly honest with how they feel. If you are an individual with low body fat, high muscle mass, and has been training to the ground, you may need this low volume-high intensity period for a **month or more.**

On the flip side, if you find yourself with higher body fat, lower muscle mass, and feel extremely energized during this phase, your taper may need to be as short as **3-7 days.** For each of these factors, **add around 1 week to your taper phase for each attribute you find yourself to fall under.**

Phase Five: Active Rest

This is the hardest phase for a driven athlete; taking a break from training. This phase takes place when the athlete has completed their competition or completed their goals. If you are really antsy to get back to training, after a few days of complete rest, you can return to light training. If the athlete is tired in any way, they should take longer rest to completely recover from a hardworking season.

Note: This periodization of phases does not just work well for weight lifting. If you are a coach looking to change up your training, follow these principles for volume and intensity and your team will prosper. If there's one thing to remember from periodization,

- Periodization is to start with high volume, but low weight on the bar.
- As the season progresses, decrease the volume and increase the weight.
- At the end of the season, increase the weight and increase the rest.

Types of Muscle Contractions

There are many ways to grow the strength and size of muscles. You can change your volume (amount of times worked out), reps/sets (# of times you lift a weight), and you can change the intensity of the lift.

When discussing the intensity of the lift, we can raise the weight and increase the contractions in your muscles

See, there are 3 main ways you can change the contractions of your muscles for a shorter, more effective workout.

The main three ways to contract your muscles are through:

1. Isometric Contractions
2. Eccentric Contractions
3. Concentric Contractions.

1. Isometric Contraction: Squeeze the Muscle

An isometric hold is where you are not moving at all, but you are holding the weight at the top or bottom of a movement, contracting your muscles in a safe way. The best example of an isometric contraction is a plank. You are holding the plank through your abdominal muscles and you are contracting them without necessarily moving them.

Fun fact: abdominal muscles respond best to this type of contraction.

2. Eccentric Contraction: Lengthen the Muscle

An eccentric contraction happens when the muscle is lengthened. This is usually when you are lowering the weight (depending on the exercise). An example of this is when you are coming down on a bicep curl. Your muscle gets lengthened at the bottom of the lift. Eccentric contractions develop the most soreness of the three contractions, meaning it is great for muscle growth, but will take longer to recover. You can perform an eccentric contraction by **lowering the weight as slow as possible.**

3. Concentric Contraction: Shorten the Muscle

A concentric contraction is the opposite of an eccentric contraction, i.e., the muscle becomes shortened. This is usually the first thing that comes to the mind of people when they hear "lifting". In our bicep example, this is where you curl the weight to the top. At some point in every lift, there will be a concentric contraction, unless you performed a set to failure.

How to Use the Three Contractions within Periodization

Back in high school, I took part in the afterschool strength and weight lifting program. It was highly effective; everyone in the sport/club gained strength on some level and most gained incredible strength and muscle. People were increasing their MAX lift by 100 and sometimes 150 pounds in just one season. After years of research involving studies and books, not to mention 9 years of lifting experience with various programs, I realized how "Coach Joe", my lifting coach, had such success with lifters of all levels. He had every set, rep, and exercise structured.

He periodized his training with high volume the first few weeks, then gradually decreased the volume towards the end of the season; so, we were well rested for max-out day (finding the most amount of weight we can lift for one rep or **"1 RM"**).

Throughout the spring season, Coach Joe would rarely have the same workout twice. If we were doing regular front squats one week, by the next week, we would implement the isometric hold to the front squat by holding the squat at the bottom of the lift for at least 3 seconds. If we were lifting upper body and doing incline bench press, we would slowly lower the weight for about 3 seconds, performing an eccentric contraction. Implementing different contractions helped us grow more muscle and in turn, strength. Before I started training properly, my maxes were as follows:

At 14-years old and no training:

Bench: 135

Back Squat: 225

Deadlift: 250

At 17-years old with 3 years of proper strength training:

Bench: 315

Back Squat: 385

Deadlift: 420

This strength increase over the course of 3-4 years has been attributed to the combination of periodization and various incorporations of muscle contractions. Without them, results would still come, but at a significantly slower rate. This is how I have been able to grow stronger and maintain my muscle mass in as little as **3 hours per week**.

The best time to incorporate variations in your lifts with contraction and periodization is **if you are stalling in your program**. Hold your squats at the bottom of the lift, lower your weights more slowly, or simply add some more reps to add variety and intensity to your training.

These contractions also work well with a partner. A partner can hold the weight against you as you raise your legs to the sky on a leg raise or apply pressure to the bar as you are curling a weight up. There's lots of room for creativity when incorporating different muscle contractions.

Another efficient way to utilize these contractions is to encompass all these techniques for a "super rep"; using each of the contractions in just one rep. To perform a super rep, lower the weight slowly, hold on the bottom, then explode on the way up; all in one rep.

Power (described below) is built from the fast rep on the way up (concentric), extra muscle tension and damage is created as the weight is lowered, and during the hold (isometric) at the bottom, there is further muscle damage. This super rep can cover the basis for most strength, size, and power goals.

Lifting For Your Goals

When an individual walks into a weight room, there should be a goal of what he/she would want to accomplish in that training session. Such goals could be: building muscle, burning fat, getting stronger, having more athletic performance, etc. Deciding on which goal you want will determine your training session. Some of these goals could overlap, while some can't (or at least not optimally in any category).

Building Muscle

If your ultimate goal is to build muscle, high volume is your best friend. This means doing 5 sets or more per exercise, with 5 or more exercises, 5 times a week. Think of 5X5X5 (sets, exercises, and frequency) as an easy reference to building muscle. Generally, more volume=more muscle, with total volume being sets x reps x frequency.

On the diet set of things, be sure you are on a caloric surplus (eating more calories than you burn). Eat around 1 gram of protein per pound of bodyweight, and eat a little more carbohydrates than usual. Creating new muscle tissue is an expensive process for your body, and it's going to be easier if you are eating enough calories. If you don't wish to use a handy app like 'MyFitnessPal', then a good rule of thumb is eat until you are full. **Be slightly fuller more often than slightly hungry** and the caloric surplus will naturally come.

If you still are still having trouble, another useful technique to find how much you need to eat (for growth), is to take your bodyweight in pounds and multiply it by 20.

Examples:

150 Pounds X 20 = 3,000 calories needed to bulk

120 Pounds X 20 = 2,400 Daily calories for bulking

Antagonist Muscles: Build More Muscle In Less Time

From observation, a great way to build muscle faster than many lifters is to train opposite or antagonist muscle groups. My favorite exercises for incorporating this style of training is with bicep curls with a rope and tricep pushdowns with a rope. The biceps and triceps are antagonistic muscle groups, meaning that as you lift one, the other stretches. As I curl up my bicep during the lift, my tricep becomes stretched and allows it to recover as I am curling. When I push down in the tricep pushdown, my bicep is being stretched. All that needs to be done is place the pin from the top of the rack to the bottom of the rack or vice versa, saving a lot of time. **Whatever muscle is being exercised/contracted, the opposite muscle is being stretched.**

Other combinations that work well with this principle are:

- **Bench Press and Pull ups**: The chest is stretched from pull ups, while the back is stretched during bench press

- **Leg Extension and Leg Curl**: The hamstrings are stretched during leg extension, while the quadriceps are stretched during leg curl.
- **Dips and Pull ups**: The dips work the lower chest and stretch the traps, while pull ups work the traps and stretch the lower chest

Another way to think about it is to **push for one exercise and then pull for another exercise.** Pulling usually involves using the back side of your body, while pushing involves muscles on the front side of your body.

Remember, this is beneficial for more muscle growth in a shorter training session, as you are performing the sets **back to back**, giving one muscle group some recovery while the opposite becomes fatigued. This greatly saves time because there is no rest when going from one exercise to the opposite exercise.

This is best used for "isolation" exercises such as most machines and "single joint" lifts, as shown in the leg extension and leg curl combo. This is because it is too fatiguing to perform supersets like these with compound movements and other multi joint exercises.

Note: Do not use this style if you only care about strength. Strength is dependent on recovery. Performing exercises back to back dampens recovery in the long term, and you will not be as strong for your compound lifts due to the fast volume build up.

Training to Muscle Failure: It isn't always necessary!

You don't want to train to failure if strength is your goal. Our definition of training to failure will be when you no longer can perform any more reps in a set, **without sacrificing form.** Training to failure heavily damages the central nervous system, dampening recovery for days or even weeks! Training to failure should not be done, especially if you are an athlete in a training program.

Remember, if strength and athletic performance is the goal, leave a few reps "in the tank" and stop your set before failure. Another problem with going to failure is that your form tends to wane and you start to bring in other muscles into the equation.

So when is the best time for failure?

The best time for training until failure in one or more sets is when you have a few days (3+) before the next time you workout (ex. Vacation, emergency, other responsibilities, etc.). This relates to the central nervous system, because you will then have some time to recover your nervous system by the time you reach your next workout.

Another scenario where training to failure is viable is if your goal is to gain muscle mass and you love pain. This is actually a decent way to gain muscle fast if you don't mind being tired occasionally and don't mind training at less than 100%.

If you are somewhere in between these scenarios and want to occasionally train to failure (which is what I like to do), **try going to failure for just the last set of any exercise in your workout.** This will give sufficient muscle damage, but not to blast your body to the ground. If you want to implement this training technique, I still recommend taking **at least one day off.**

Other Goals

Burning Fat

If your goal is to burn off more fat, you want to be sure to optimize not only your training, but also your diet. Burning fat and dieting are not always for aesthetic reasons. Sometimes an athlete will benefit from some weight loss to fit a competition weight that will feel best for them. An endurance runner will not want to be carrying an extra 10 pounds of fat when they are running over 26 miles; they will (most likely) feel and perform better when they lose the extra 10 pounds.

On the training side of discussion, the goal is to maintain muscle while losing fat. This is not only because muscle is jet fuel for one's metabolism, but also because muscle is a great driver of athletic performance.

The best way to maintain muscle is through consistent training and getting enough protein. To be on the safe side, get around 1 gram of protein per pound of bodyweight (ex. 160 lbs = 160 g of protein). This will ensure you hold on to your athletic performance while simultaneously reaching a comfortable competition weight.

While you may be able to build muscle without being in a caloric surplus all the time, you **absolutely** have to be in a caloric deficit to lose fat. This caloric deficit will force you to sacrifice volume, because energy levels are much lower during a caloric deficit.

Sets should stay around the number 5, with the exercises staying around 5 as well, but only *if* you lower the days per week to as low as 3 days per week. **Something in terms of volume should be sacrificed** the longer you stay in a caloric deficit, with the consequences being extreme burnout. If you are looking for a simple formula that is fairly accurate, take your bodyweight in pounds and multiply by 10.

For example, if you are 200 pounds, 2,000 calories will be a great starting point to shed some fat. Burning fat is a massive topic that can become extremely complicated under different conditions, so stay focused and **keep lifting and getting your protein.**

Building Muscle and Burning Fat at the same time: Can you do it?

There is a small fraction of the lifting community that could burn fat and build muscle simultaneously. The best candidates for this position are those that have just started lifting, those that have not lifted in a few months, genetic freaks, and those on steroids. The reason these populations could simultaneously burn fat and build muscle is because their muscle building response is so great; they could build muscle in a calorie deficit.

Remember This: A caloric surplus simply **helps** muscle building, while a caloric deficit is a **requirement** for fat loss. Training is the biggest driver in muscle gaining. And while training helps fat loss, you can overeat the calories you burned through training with just a few hundred calories (3 pieces of fruit) and undo your fat loss efforts.

Modified Reverse Pyramid Training: A Program for Strength

When my ultimate goal is to achieve strength with a little bit of muscle growth on the back end, I implement my own version on reverse pyramid training. Here's an example first with an explanation after.

Bench Press (or any **compound** movement):

Set 1 (warm up): 20X135

Rest: 30 s

Set 2 (Heaviest): 3X275

Rest: Unlimited

Set 3 (2nd Heaviest): 4X260

Rest: 3-5 minutes

Set 4 (3rd Heaviest): 5X250

Rest: 1-2 minutes

Set 5: 8X225

Do you see what is happening here? After a quick warm up set, I immediately start with my heaviest set. This will focus on my type 2 muscle fibers or "fast twitch" muscle fibers to grow strength, speed, and a little bit of size. As I go through more sets, I increased the reps and lower the weight, hence the "reverse pyramid" part. By the time I am on my last set, in this case set 5, I am less focused on strength and more focused on muscle contractions; feeling the mind connect with the muscle.

This is further exemplified with **the rest decreasing throughout the sets, giving the muscles less time to recover and in turn, more muscle in less time.** This is why it's a "modified" reverse period because most reverse pyramid training programs do not incorporate strength.

Lifting for Strength and Power

Lifting for strength and lifting for power are similar in some ways and different in others. Strength training is focused on lifting as much weight as possible in any way possible while power training is more finessed. Power training needs to be incorporated for all athletes *on some level,* as it is what will increase the **explosiveness** of the athlete. However, explosive movements can be implemented to almost any lift or bodyweight movement to turn it into power training. For example, you could take the back squat:

Strength Styled Sets:

5 sets of 3 reps at 80% of 1RM

Power Styled Sets:

5 sets of 8 reps at 60% of 1RM- **with a jump**

Here is a chart that can help distinguish the two:

Strength vs. Power Training Properties

Strength Training	Power Training
Overcoming resistance	Overcoming resistance
Heavy weight (75%+ of 1RM)	Any weight
Contributes some muscle gain	Lifting **as fast** as possible
Moving **from point A to B** the easiest way	Plyometrics and other body weight exercises benefit

Optimizing Your Performance: "Hacks", Tips, and Tricks

How to Breathe During Exercise: Understanding which part of your breath is best for each point in your lift

Scientific research has shown that strength increases by about 5% when you clench your teeth, when you clench your fists, and when you know how to breath.

Knowing how to breathe during your lift would take your strength to the next level. Did you know that you are strongest when your breath is held, a little weaker when you exhale, and are at your weakest when you inhale?

This means at the **bottom** of your lifting movement (ex. Bottom of a squat, the bar touching your chest on bench press, etc.), you want to **hold your breath**. This is because you are naturally your weakest at this low point so you have to compensate by holding your breath. **As you come up** from the lift, the bar feels lighter and lighter, so **exhaling your breath is the most beneficial**. As you come down in the movement of your lift, you should inhale so as to prepare for holding your breath as the lift becomes harder and harder.

As a quick summary, **remember this:**

- You are strongest when you hold your breath
- You are a little weaker when you exhale
- You are weakest when you inhale

Give this a try right now! Take a deep breath and hold it... Don't you feel powerful and strong? That is how you will feel underneath the bar. Now exhale. What did you feel? You may have experienced your body relaxing as you exhale. Pay attention to your breath from time to time. **You will discover that it is a huge factor in many daily activities** in decreasing stress, falling asleep faster and deeper, and ultimately being in control of your day.

Warming Up: It's not just to get you tired

I used to think that the more I warmed up, the more tired I was going to be during the main training portion; so, I admittedly didn't warm up well with my teams. Most people know the importance of warming up and how great it is for optimizing performance, but I was too stubborn to actually try to properly warm up Since then, I have researched and experimented many times over, with and without warming up and how my performance responded to it.

The internal temperature of your muscles can greatly affect your performance. Did you know that for every 2 degrees Farenheit your internal temperature is raised, your body can become up to 7% stronger? This is because the mitochondria in your muscles perform best when your body is just a few degrees above its normal state.

If you're not carrying around a thermometer like most people, the best way to know you finished warming up is when you have just **started to break a sweat**. At this point, your body is primed for optimal performance at its best body temperature without getting yourself fatigued.

Nitric Oxide

Another reason warming up will enhance your performance is blood flow. When your body has more blood flow, your body creates something called nitric oxide. This is a very **good** thing. **Nitric oxide** expands the blood vessels, increases blood flow, decreases plaque growth, increases blood clotting, and opens your muscles to intake more nutrients. So if you want to get the most benefits and nutrients from your food, be sure to warm up at least until you break a sweat.

Breathing through your nose is another easy and simple way to boost nitric oxide. The next time you warm up, **try to**

perform all or most of the warm up by only breathing through your nose. Give this tip a try while you are walking somewhere or doing anything. This will boost the overall oxygen in your blood over time in a natural way.

There are some foods that can boost nitric oxide. Here's a list to add to your grocery cart:

- Watermelon
- Bananas
- Spinach
- Seafood
- Garlic
- Dark Chocolate (the darker the better)
- Lemons
- Grapefruit
- Walnuts
- Oranges
- Rhubarb
- Apples
- Strawberries
- Beets

Fun Fact: Beets are my favorite food to boost nitric oxide naturally in the body.

Sleep: Sometimes doing nothing is better than doing something

Have you ever had to wake up early in the morning day after day for school, work, or sports? As a hardworking lifter, athlete, or both, you deserve your sleep. In fact, you should make sleep a priority, especially as you progress further into your training.

The longer and deeper you sleep, the more Growth Hormone (GH) you will release. Growth Hormone is the ultimate anti-aging hormone, destroying inflammatory free radicals that are created from stress and exercise. This means you are literally slowing down time (in terms of your body) the more that you sleep by increasing how long you can live. Growth Hormone will also help grow healthy hair, skin, and nails; it isn't called "beauty sleep" for nothing.

Rest is just as important as training. However, this does not mean that you should sleep 12 hours a day or sit on the couch for hours. Rest compliments training just as training complements resting. The more you train, the more rest you need to compensate for training; like a teeter totter. Rest is where the adaptations and growth occur *from* your training.

Sadly, most people do *not* rest enough and become burnt out and quit their activity.

The best way to get deeper, more restful sleep is to have a sleeping mask. The sleeping mask will create a dark (almost black) atmosphere in almost any environment. This dark environment helps your body produce melatonin; your main sleep hormone. This happens extremely fast and your mind will wander less and less. This saves hours of tossing and turning and will get you to sleep faster so you can take on your next day of training with full energy.

Training Template: Strength

Shown below is a great training template that can be mixed and matched with the list of exercises (further below).

Lower Body

Exercise	Sets	Reps	Rest	Intensity/ Weight
Deadlift	3	4	Unlimited	High
Step ups (weighted)	4	6/Leg	90 s	Med-High
Squat Jumps	3	8	60 s	BW
Bulgarian Split Squat	3	5/Leg	90 s	High
Plank	2	90 sec	30 s	BW

Upper Body

Exercise	Sets	Reps	Rest	Intensity/ Weight
Bench Press	5	5	60-120 s	High
BB Bent Over Row	4	6	90 s	Med-High
Shoulder Press	3	6	60 s	High
Lying Triceps Extension	3	5/Arm	90 s	High
Clap Push ups (knees if starting out)	3	6	45 s	BW and ALL OUT

Note: If you are focusing on strength, you need to decrease the reps and sets but increase the weight. The 'rest' noted in this section is extremely variable, since everyone is in a different cardiovascular condition. It is advised to remember that when training for strength, you are to rest until you feel almost at 100% energy. Don't go into a set, breathing heavily with an extremely high heart rate; it will defeat the purpose of the workout.

Training Template: Muscle Growth

Lower Body

Exercise	Sets	Reps	Rest	Intensity/ Weight
Back Squat	5	6	60-90 s	Med-High
BB Single Leg Squat	4	8/Leg	60 s	Med-High
DB Calf Raises	5	20	30 s	Med
DB Lunge	3	8/Leg	90 s	Med-High
Wall Sit	2	90 sec TUT	60 s	BW

Upper Body

Exercise	Sets	Reps	Rest	Intensity/ Weight
Incline Bench Press	5	8	60-90 s	Med-High
Pull Ups	5	8	60 s	Med-High
DB Curls	4	8/Arm	60 s	Med
DB Shrugs	3	20	30 s	Med
Bicycles	3	60 s TUT	30 s	BW+Contract hard

Note:

If your goal is to gain physical muscle size, volume is key. Focus on contracting and *feeling* the muscles and you will reach your optimal size before you know it.

Training Template: Power Training Exercises

Full Body

Exercise	Sets	Reps	Rest	Intensity/ Weight
Power Clean	5	4	Unlimited	Med-High
Standing Shoulder Press	4	6	90 s	Med
Good Morning	4	8	30 s	Low-Med
Box Jumps	3	8	60 s	High
Medicine Ball Throws	2	6	30 s	Med-High
Battle Ropes	2	30sec TUT	90 s	All Out

Note: Power cleans are amazing for building speed, power, and explosion. It is **horrible** for muscle growth since the eccentric and isometric portions are almost nonexistent.

List of Weight Lifting Exercises and their Benefits

The templates above are just general guidelines to follow and the exercises are not as important as the volume and intensity associated with them. Feel free to mix the template with any of the exercises shown below for your desired goal. My notes following the exercise are the way I use the exercise, but you can manipulate the volume and intensity for your goals.

Chest

- **Incline Barbell Bench Press**- Great for gaining general strength and some upper chest development
- **Flat Barbell Bench Press**- Great for gaining strength and mid-chest development

- **Incline Dumbbell Press**- Great for growing muscle in the upper chest and evening out the strength in your arms
- **Flat Dumbbell Bench**- Evening out strength in arms to create more balance and strength for the Barbell bench press
- **Dips**- Developing the lower chest and rarely used for strength
- **Cable Crossovers**- Development of the inner chest
- **Incline Chest flys**- Great for development of the upper chest
- **Medicine Ball Throws**- Builds power and recruits fast twitch muscle fibers in the chest

Shoulders

- ***BB Shoulder Press (standing)-** Best compound movement for the growth of shoulders with additional use of the abs and back for stabilizing the body
- **BB Shoulder Press (sitting)-** Higher weight can be used for more strength of the shoulders since you don't have to stabilize your body
- **Seated Dumbbell Press**- Evening out strength and size of shoulders
- **Dumbbell Lateral Raise**- Developing the outside of your shoulders, getting heavier towards the top of the movement

- ***Cable Lateral Raise-** Similar to the dumbbell version, but a constant linear tension throughout the movement
- **Face Pull-** Developing the trapezius and upper back muscles
- **Dumbbell Front Raise-** Developing and growing the front of the shoulders (*Usually this muscle group is not a problem for most people as it tends to get overdeveloped through incline and flat bench press)

Back

- **Barbell Deadlift-** Great for total body strength, athletic performance, and overall muscle development (*lengthy in set up and tear down of weights)
- **Barbell Row-** Great for developing thickness in the back
- **Dumbbell row-** Great for evening out the strength and size of the back muscles
- **Pull Ups-** Best all-around exercise for the back for strength and size. Wide grip for more lat development and close grip for more focus on shoulders
- ***Chin ups-** The only compound movement for your biceps
- **Lat Pulldown-** Great for working on just the lats
- **Shrugs (BB or DB)-** Great exercise for the traps

Abdominals (Abs)

- **Planks**- Implementing the isometric hold
- *__Bicycles__*- Fast breakdown of your abs and my favorite exercise to get in a good exercise in a short amount of time
- **Leg Lifts**- This could be done on many pull up machines as well. Targets the lower abs.
- **Russian/Roman Twist**- Works the serratus (upper side abs), especially when weight is used.
- **Incline Sit Ups-** A great total ab contraction through extra range of motion compared to traditional ab exercises

Legs

- *__BB Back Squat__*- Best "bang for your buck" lower body exercise for strength and development of your hamstrings (backside of thigh)
- *__BB Front Squat__*- Another great lower body exercise for development of your quadriceps (front of thigh)
- **Leg Press**- Best machine for pain free squatting that is great for starters, taller people, or people with rough joints in pain
- *__Lunge (BW, DB, or BB)__*- Great compound movement for development of the legs that can be done anywhere

- **Leg Extension**- Machine great for quads (be sure not to go too heavy or you may have joint issues)
- **Leg Curl**- Machine great for your hamstrings
- **Box Jumps**- Builds power in the legs

Arms

- **BB Curl**- Best curling exercise for strength
- ***E. Z. Bar Curl**- The jagged bar helps with keeping your joints comfortable with full range of motion
- **DB Curl**- Great for general bicep development
- **Hammer Curl**- Great for developing the length of your bicep (front part)
- ***BB Close Grip Bench Press**- Great for developing the triceps and inner chest and is the best compound movement for your arms
- ***Triceps Pushdown (rope)**- A great exercise for developing mass in your triceps (back of arms) that has a constant tension that is equal throughout the lift
- ***Bicep curl (rope)**- Great for immediately after the tricep pushdown as an antagonist muscle (see above) and for constant linear tension for even development over other curl-type exercises
- **Battle Ropes**- Great explosive work for the arms. Great cardio for longer periods.

Notes:

favorite of mine = *

DB= Dumbbells

BB= Barbells

If you noticed some trends from the exercise list, **the most important things to remember are:**

1. **Barbells:** Focus on **strength**
2. **Dumbbells: Evening out strength** on both sides of your body

Cables and Ropes: Focus on **muscle growth**

Tools and Supplements

There are a few main supplements that help sports performance. Most other supplements are usually a waste of time as they are either filled with banned ingredients, don't work at all, or can actually hurt you. These supplements are the safest and develiver the best "bang for your buck" that could help sports performance.

Creatine Monohydrate

Creatine is naturally produced by the body but you can also get it through your food. Some foods that contain creatine are shrimp, beef, chicken, and most other types of meats. You can also get creatine in supplement form which is the form of creatine that is most practical for noticing a difference in performance.

Creatine helps your performance by allowing water (and other nutrients) to rush into the muscle cells and swell up. This allows for greater strength and speed for lifting and high intensity sports. Sadly, some people are non-responders to creatine, so it's important to check to see if creatine will even work for you. You can start with a dose of **about 5 grams per day,** which is usually just a teaspoon from most supplement bottles. If you are noticing a bit more strength in the next few weeks, you respond well to creatine. Stick with creatine monohydrate, as it is the most researched supplement among the supplement industry

Whey Protein

Another great supplement for your performances is whey protein. Remember, I mentioned earlier that you should get one gram of protein per pound of body weight? Whey protein could help you here.

There are 3 main types of whey protein:

1. Isolate
2. Concentrate
3. Hydrolysate

1. Isolate: This contains 90+% protein by weight, with low fats and low carbs and lactose removed and moderately priced.

2. Concentrate: This contains 30-90% protein by weight with the rest being carbs and fats.

3. Hydrolysate: This contains extremely broken down protein that is extremely digestible but is the most expensive

All of these different types of protein will help your lifting and athletic performance by helping you achieve that 1 gram of protein per pound of body weight recommendation. If you want the best bang for your buck, concentrates and isolates will be the best options for you, as they are cheaper than hydrolysate.

If you tend to have an upset stomach (from isolate, concentrate, or just in general), whey hydrolysate will be your solution. Protein will be the best tool to help your muscles recover and grow back stronger. Think of whey protein as convenient protein to be used to *supplement* your protein needs when you can't or don't want to cook.

Coffee/Caffeine

I am a huge fan of coffee. There's something about it that just puts me in a great mood along with a motivating feeling to do more work each day. I also use coffee for sport and lifting performance. Caffeine is a stimulant that affects the nervous system. Remember when we were discussing the nervous system breaking down when training to failure? The nervous system breaks down if it becomes extremely overtaxed, with a recovery period long enough to drain your energy for days to even weeks. Reasons for a corrupted nervous system are overtraining, too much stress, not enough sleep, and too much caffeine.

So why have I recommended coffee? Doesn't coffee contain caffeine? In times like this, it's always good to remember, the dose of something determines the *poison* of something. Caffeine in high amounts will make you feel as I like to say, "Wired and tired," so, we need to find the correct dosage for ourselves. To test your tolerance, take 1 cup at a time each day and find the point where you have a moderate amount of energy without your heart beating out of your chest. What I find is best for lifting is no more than 1 cup of coffee, but what works best for me may not work best for you, since I have a weak tolerance.

If you don't like coffee, you could try pre workout supplements or energy drinks. However, they are a slippery slope because your body quickly adapts and then depends on them *just to feel normal.* I'd recommend mixing only a small amount in your water bottle, so you are mostly hydrating yourself; getting a smaller kick of caffeine in the background.

If you just have this light dose of caffeine, you are stimulating your nervous system just enough to simulate the "fight or flight" response in your body to move with maximum power and speed; something that will greatly help your lifting.

If there's one thing to remember from consuming caffeine to help your performance; **smaller is better**. You should rely on your training, nutrition, and a good warmup as your base for performance. Drink 1-2 cups of coffee to *supplement* your training.

Fun Fact: Caffeine is a banned substance by the NCAA, but only in an amount of about 8 cups (600-1,000 mg of caffeine) of coffee consumed around 2 hours before competition. This is why a pre-workout supplement is not a great idea, due to caffeine content upwards of 240 mg per serving. You wouldn't want that amount of caffeine anyways as it does not help performance and could give the user a heart attack during exercise.

MCT Oil

MCT oil is a supplement but almost considered not a supplement. MCTs or "medium chain triglycerides" can be found in coconut oil, which means it is part-food. "Triglyceride" basically means just fat; the only macronutrient in MCT oil. However, MCT oil itself is a supplement because it is usually extracted from coconut oil or manufactured in a lab.

MCT oil is a great energy source for activities that are in the mid-distance range where the time a person is exercising is between 30 and 60 seconds. As in the name, it is a medium chain triglyceride, not a short or long chain triglyceride like butter or other fats. This fat bypasses the liver when eating, meaning it almost instantaneously gives you energy. Just 1 tablespoon will produce a burst of stable energy lasting around 1-4 hours.

If you are nervous about trying MCT oil, give coconut oil a try! It has around 40% MCT oil in it, along with health benefits of "lauric acid" to help with inflammation and recovery from workouts. I'm no coconut oil guru, but I have found coconut oil and MCT oil helps me generally feel great. For training, there tends to be noticeable boost of **endurance.**

Energy Sources During a Set

When you are lifting and performing a set, your body is using different types of fuel as the intensity or reps are manipulated. The energy system corresponding with the reps below being **only accurate if the last rep is failure or 1-2 reps shy of failure.**

Reps 1-3: You are using the creatine phosphate system

Reps 4-15: You are using the anaerobic system

Reps 15+: You are using the aerobic system

The Creatine Phosphate System

Earlier, I mention creatine as a supplement for increasing speed and strength. The creatine phosphate system is the reason creatine gets a shout out. During the first few seconds of any intense exercise, in this case reps 1-3, you are **using your creatine stores.** Earlier, I mentioned that there are some foods that contain creatine such as meat and seafood. While these foods do replenish your creatine stores, you can't always keep up with the demand. This is where supplementation comes in if you want to train hard and recover hard.

Fun fact: Usually the first hard and fast movement you do anytime and anywhere involves creatine and its phosphate system.

The Anaerobic System

In a rep range of 4-15, you are starting to tap into your anaerobic system. This system is also used in sprinting. For the anaerobic system, "time under tension" (TUT) or time you are exercising is around 15 seconds up to a minute. At this intensity, a great amount of sugar (glucose/carbohydrate) is being used, so go ahead and allow more carbohydrates in the diet. A great sport that utilizes the anaerobic system is American football, sprinting on and off in repeated intervals. You will use this energy system the most when lifting

Remember: Think of any intense movement that lasts longer than 10 seconds as you using your anaerobic system and eat more carbohydrates.

The Aerobic System

At 15 or more reps (or TUT over around 1 minute), you are using the aerobic system. As the distance in an endurance event increases, you are forced to use more of your aerobic system, because the lower intensity needs to be maintained longer . At this intensity, contrary to popular belief, fat is your best friend. Fat is your friend when you go the distance (or do lots of reps) because of fat being slow digesting, giving a steady state energy longer than the crash carbs provide.

Notes: For more information on energy sources, intensities, and even body types, check out my other book, *Optimization For Athletes: Macronutrient Edition* here on Amazon:

(http://a.co/d/9hGoDdd)

Closing Thoughts

Spread the word about this information as it is not commonly told to people. Many athletes and average gym goers (which are athletes) do not go into weight lifting with their goals in mind, aimlessly getting in a "work out". Apply the training styles and training tips laid out in this book and you will achieve strength, athletic performance, and muscle mass faster than the competition.

If you have received value from this book, leave a comment and a rating! For more feedback or questions, email me through my business email: breheimgregory@gmail.com

This is my 2nd book and I hope to learn what was good or bad and what to work on so that it could be improved on in subsequent future writings. I would also like to hear what you would like to know. Take the next step and use this knowledge into your next competitive season and optimize your performance!

About the Author

Greg has participated in a variety of sports and worked with many athletes at many different sports clinics in swimming, weightlifting, football, and track and field. Having competed in numerous weight lifting tournaments, Greg is also a swim coach for the St. Croix Swim Club (2018), one of the most competitive clubs in the midwest. He is a huge fan of trial and error to find some of the best techniques for optimization for each given scenario, constantly learning at each opportunity.